Latch On To Success: Empowering You On Your Breastfeeding Journey

Deborah Bowers-Street

THE BREASTFEEDING ACADEMY

DEDICATION

This book is for you...... I see you, I hear you. Overwhelmed with all of the information out there – should I breastfeed, bottle feed, pump, time feeds, not time feeds, store breast milk, top up with formula....argh!

I *was* you. And now I am here to help you, and to empower you to have the breastfeeding journey that *you* want.

* * * * *

And to my beautiful babies – thank you all for being such truly wonderful and remarkable people! You all make me so proud every single day.

"I love you the whole universe"

"Pooh bums"

Latch On To Success

Latch On To Success

CONTENTS

Latch On To Success

Latch On To Success

AUTHOR'S NOTE

The title took me a long time to decide on ~ I wanted to create an informative book, but one that also enables women to feel *empowered* with their breastfeeding journey.

Having breastfed seven children myself, I have experienced first hand that overwhelming feeling of not knowing what I was doing, feeling I was doing it all wrong. Then when I did feel I was getting it right, I thought my milk had dried up.

It was only on baby *number seven* that I educated myself and oh how I wish I knew back then what I know now.

So this book has been written from a place of guidance, love and *no* judgement. What is right for you is right for you. I just want to give you the tools to make an informed choice

~ D ~

1

(HOW MANY BABIES?)

Congratulations! Whether you are newly pregnant, close to your due date, a first-time parent, or a 7th time parent, you are obviously here as you wish to breastfeed your baby.

One of the first things for you to remember is that knowing how to breastfeed is not knowledge that you are born with, more a skill that you learn. It is a skill to develop, a technique, and knowing this from the start is a key step to your success.

The second thing to know is that breastfeeding is natural. It is not sexual. It is recommended, and is not just beneficial for the baby, but for the mother too. The World Health Organisation (WHO) recommends breastfeeding to the minimum age of 2 years old. MINIMUM! So many people have the opinion that nursing your baby beyond 6 months is "just for the benefit of the mother", or "she just doesn't want to let her baby grow up". But no! This ongoing narrative needs to change. In fact, nursing your baby on demand, and holding your baby on demand, helps to make them more independent, and creates a nurturing bond between you.

When put that way, doesn't it make more sense? Their wants and needs are met, they know that you are there for them when needed, and therefore feel safer to take these small steps away from you as they get older.

Back in the 1960's, formula companies allegedly paid staff to dress as nurses to promote formula within the labour wards. This kind of subtle advertising has led us to a society that views breastfeeding as only a sexual thing. Breastfeeding women get asked to cover up in restaurants or cafes, asked to feed their baby in the toilet. Yet those same people likely don't think twice about breasts on show at the beach!

So let's change that shall we? We are a generation of strong women, and together we can help people to become informed about breastfeeding and build each other up.

Before we start, it should just be mentioned that the information offered in this eBook does not include the use of drugs, or mechanical inventions, such as the use of nipple shields, or the regular use of bottles. The main purpose is to show you the basics of breastfeeding, which require only you and your baby.

A great way to get the most out of this eBook is to show it to your partner, parents, whoever is in your support system.

Sometimes we end up so close to the problem that we cannot see it for ourselves. Having people to support you can be key to your breastfeeding journey. Some of what you read may contradict what you already know, and what others know. But it will help you to avoid that conflicting advice.

Before we begin, I want to offer you some insight into my own breastfeeding journey.

I am a mother to 7 beautiful babies, ranging from (at the time of writing in 2023) 19 years down to 2 and a half years old. I will add here that all 7 babies were vaginal births (breastfeeding after a caesarean section can be slightly different), with no pain relief for 2 babies, gas and air only for 2 babies, 2 water births (1 with gas and air, 1 without), and one with an epidural (the last baby!)

Baby #1, I was told by my midwife in the follow up checks that I was to maintain a strict 4 hour breastfeeding pattern. She would cry around 2 hours after a feed, and so I introduced a dummy very early on, which would settle her for a while longer. At 4 months old she didn't seem to be getting enough milk from me, and so I started to wean her onto baby rice. She was also waking a lot during the night and so I moved her onto bottles (thinking that my milk wasn't enough). That first time, she drank 2 x 9oz bottles – and promptly threw it all back up. I also gave her the thicker hungry baby formula at night. I now know that around 3-4 months is a key growth spurt, and that most babies have a 4 month sleep regression!

Baby #2. At 3 weeks old I started to spend anywhere between 2 to 3 hours an evening feeding her, from one breast entirely, to the other, and back again. It was exhausting. My older child was just 21 months old, and I felt like I was just doing it all wrong. I considered giving her a bottle, but I was told that I couldn't combine breast feeding and formula feeding. So I gave up feeding her at just 3 weeks old. Again, the first growth spurt is between 2 to 3 weeks.

Baby #3, was born when Baby #1 was 3 years old, and Baby#2 was just 17 months. But he actually fed very well until he was 10 months old. My periods hadn't returned at that stage and we knew that we wanted to have another baby. So I stopped feeding him and promptly fell pregnant with Baby #4.

Baby #4. She was fed exclusively by the breast until she was 4 months old, maybe even 5 or 6 months. During a health visitor visit, she was weighed and measured on the 9th centile on her growth chart. She was a dinky little tot! But was 8 lb 13 Oz when born, so not tiny. I was advised to switch to formula. She is now 14 years old, 5 foot 8 inches tall, and a UK size 6. She was always going to be a smaller build! It is worth noting that I am 5' 8", and her father is 6'. But these weren't factors taken into consideration on growth charts.

Baby #5. Again, fed until that 4-month growth spurt, where I thought that I wasn't producing enough milk for her.

Baby #6. I felt that I finally got it right! She was fed to 13 months, where I stopped as it felt that she was 'too old' for breastfeeding. I was pulled into the expectations of society, and that to continue to feed her myself was wrong. She moved straight on to cow's milk.

Baby #7. Well.....we are 2 and a half years in, and still going strong. My initial plan was to get to the first 6 months, and then see how it went. At 8 months old she accidentally bit me. I was so upset. I tried filling her up with food to get her back to sleep that night, and she simply needed me. I worked through it that night (she had cut my nipple), and the next day we went shopping for formula and bottles. But she wouldn't touch it! So we continued with breastfeeding. She is quite an active child, and sitting to nurse gives her so much comfort, and enables us both to sit quietly and spend quality time together. I am truly grateful for the time that I get to spend with her.

Yes it means that I am the one to get her to sleep for naps and for bedtime, yes I'm the one to settle her back to sleep at night (but we co-sleep so this isn't an issue anyway. We followed the guidelines from The Lullaby Trust from birth and it has been amazing, and has helped us to keep our sanity in those early days). But I wouldn't change it. I've no idea how long this nursing stage will last for, but I do see daily how happy and how independent she is becoming.

2

CHOOSING TO BREASTFEED OR BOTTLE FEED

Evidence shows us that breastfeeding truly IS best for babies. And actually, best for mothers too, especially in those first post-natal days, encouraging your womb to shrink back down to the original size.

What many people don't understand is that:

1 – Breast milk is perfectly balanced for babies. It contains precisely the right amount of carbohydrates, fat, protein and minerals.

2 – Breastmilk changes composition during not only the day, but even during the feed, to meet the needs of a baby. This composition changes as the baby grows.

Breastfeeding is also best for women too (we are not talking here about women who suffer from Post-Natal Depression, or who find that they struggle to feed their baby). In breastfeeding, their physical and emotional welfare are connected. It forms part of the 4th trimester also, where the baby needs to remain with their mother.

Women who breastfeed their baby should find that:

- their wombs contract more quickly after birth
- the blood lost after childbirth flows faster and is completed more quickly
- they are less likely to become pregnant again soon after birth (not a reliable method of contraception however!)
- the hormones that they secrete while breastfeeding make them feel calm
- they tend to (not always though) lose weight more easily, as their body uses stored energy, meaning that the mother doesn't need to 'eat for two'.

Breastfeeding is far more than just a way to feed a baby. Babies respond to the skin-to-skin that occurs. Crying and distressed babies can be comforted by the physical contact. It can be a lovely way to sit and spend time with an older child too. These positive feelings of nurturing and closeness can help to create a wonderful foundation for a mother-baby relationship. Building confidence and self-esteem for them both.

Breastfeeding well can help a woman to gain confidence in her role as a mother, and this must be helped as much as possible.

Choosing Whether To Breastfeed Or Bottle Feed

For each woman, this decision is often an emotional one. There are many factors that she will consider, which may sometimes cause conflict, and which can be added to by stories of negativity from other people. Perhaps they struggled to breastfeed their own baby, perhaps their baby didn't put on weight, perhaps their baby struggled to latch, perhaps they received criticism for feeding in public. Perhaps you know that you'll need to return to work after the baby is born? Or maybe you want to share the responsibility of feeding your baby with your partner, so bottles seem like the only option?

It is so important to talk these feelings through if you can. Family members can bond in so many other wonderful ways, not just by feeding them a bottle. Think about what is best for you, about how you feel. Make a note of your worries. Share these with your midwife or health visitor. In the meantime, the best thing that you can do is educate yourself: learn as much as you can in advance, speak to people about your wish to breastfeed and how they can support you.

Breastfeeding when returning to work can be a tough subject for many women. For some, returning to work soon after the birth may be their plan. Every woman's definition of 'soon' will differ, however. For some, this may be a few weeks, for others it might not be until their child starts school. Which might pose the question of whether a mother should breastfeed at all?

Remember that breastfeeding is better for both of you, even if it is for a short time, and is better than not breastfeeding at all.

The more time that you spend with your baby during the first few weeks and months, the better for you both. The best preparation for going back to work is to be breastfeeding without problems. To return while potentially having issues, could cause further issues in your breastfeeding journey. It is worth speaking to your

employer to find out how they can support breastfeeding

mothers. It might be that you breastfeed in the morning and evenings, and your baby is given expressed milk in a bottle during the day. You might be able to express at work (and your work should give you a private space to do so). Someone may be able to bring you your baby during the day for feeds.

Choosing to Breastfeed

While most women do know that choosing to breastfeed is best for the baby (and them), a lot of women choose not to from the start or choose to stop after a short time. Their reasons are their own and valid and should be supported.

Some reasons might include:

- Feeling that breastfeeding is distasteful
- Early trauma in her own life
- Believing that bottles are more convenient
- Believing that bottle fed babies sleep better
- Believing that offering bottles may help family members to bond with the baby
- Believing that formula milk is better than breast milk
- Pain due to incorrect latching
- Pain due to tongue tie in the baby

- Baby fussing at the breast, causing everyone to think that the mother isn't producing enough milk

It is important that you make your own free choice, from your own reading and research, coupled with your own gut feelings. If you have the full facts available to you on both breastfeeding, bottle feeding, breast milk and artificial milk, this should help you to decide.

Women are often prevented from doing what they would like to do by:

- _Misinformation_ given by others, with their own thoughts, experiences and assumptions
- _Lack of skilled support_, especially in the first few weeks. This is often not helped in societies where breastfeeding figures are low
- _Practical difficulties_ that they can't solve

A huge amount of breastfeeding misinformation comes from social causes. The advertising from the formula companies, the bottle manufacturers and the pram makers. This isn't helped when these views are also held by partners, mothers, grandmothers, in-laws. Or by other people being 'put out' by your breastfeeding.

Please do not feel guilty if you find yourself wanting to avoid conflict.

You can see how it happens though.... all it takes is a baby that seems unhappy, with a new mother who feels unsure of the best way to care for her baby (and with little support), with the demands of new-found tiredness.

And this creates the perfect recipe for breastfeeding failure.

ADD to this that information is often misinformation, how so many people feel uncomfortable seeing a woman breastfeeding her baby, and the problem continues to spread far and wide.

But we can change this..... this change can start with you.... and the ripples can continue through your family, friends, your own children and grandchildren.

3

BREASTFEEDING SUPPORT

Before you begin your breastfeeding journey, try to find some breastfeeding support. This may be in the form of a post-natal doula, breastfeeding counsellor, breastfeeding support group, a family member or friend with breastfeeding experience with their own children. They can not only support you on your breastfeeding path but could offer you some much needed rest. Try to choose your helpers before the baby is born.

Note: even if you do not have a good support network, this does NOT mean that you will fail. Many women bring up their babies single-handedly and are very successful at doing so!

You will need three things from your support/helpers:

- *Good emotional support* especially on those days when tiredness and feeding feel overwhelming
- *Real practical help* with household tasks, including shopping, cleaning, caring for older children
- *Skilled assistance* if you have difficulty or if you develop problems

Before you ask someone for help (especially those who are not professionally chosen by you), make sure that they are as interested in breastfeeding as you. Someone who doesn't agree with breastfeeding, or is uncomfortable with seeing it, is not the kind of support person that you need. Someone who is kind, supportive and willing to not only be asked, but to see when you need help can be invaluable.

Some common groups for support include:

- La Leche League
- The Breastfeeding Network
- The Association of Breastfeeding Mothers

Support from your partner

Your partner can also be a wonderful support for breastfeeding. While many may find the idea makes them feel uncomfortable to start with, likely to be because breasts are so sexualised, you might find that they come round to the idea of breastfeeding quickly. They will likely be able to see the benefits to both you and the baby and be fully supportive.

Some partners may wish for you to express, or move the baby on to formula, so that they can bond with the baby. However, there are so many other ways for them to bond. Skin to skin cuddles, bath time, playing, can all create a wonderful and unique bond, just between them. In the same way that you are bonding with your baby, so can they, just in a different way.

It will help you on your journey tremendously that if you have a partner, that they are on board with you breastfeeding. Let them read this guide, let them research for themselves, and understand that even with possible cultural issues, breastfeeding is by far the best thing for you and your baby. In the long run, it will also be better for your partner, as the baby you now have together will be healthier, and family relationships will be better and stronger.

Many will hope that you will express in the early days for them to give a bottle or suggest a bottle of formula for them to feed to the baby. Please understand that doing this in the early weeks of the life of the baby and your breastfeeding journey could undermine the success of breastfeeding. I am sure that if many knew that artificial milk is not as good for the baby as breast milk, that a lot more partners would encourage the breastfeeding journey for you and your baby.

Your partner can have a key role in those early days, weeks, and months, that will help you all to create a wonderful nurturing bond.

They can do this by:

- Giving you love and support in your desire to breastfeed
- Be attentive to what you need
- Listen when you ask them for something that will support you (even if only a glass of water)
- Take over the running of the household, including meals and childcare of older children
- Keep unwanted visitors at bay until you are ready
- Keeping you comfortable, including offering extra cushions, giving you a massage, leaving you to sleep when you need to

It is important though to make sure that if you need support that isn't obvious, that you ask. No one is a mind reader. They might not realise that you would LOVE to take a shower, and not think to take the baby to enable you to do so. So please do express what you need help with. This can help relationships in so many ways.

And TALK. Try to set aside some time each day to both talk

through how you are both feeling. This time can take an incredible toll on relationships, and communication is always key.

Taking Care of Yourself

You might have expected to be sore, and tired. But perhaps not realised *quite* how much. Self-care is so important in general, but even more so during this period. Make sure that you set aside some time for yourself each day.... even if only 5 minutes to sit in the garden, or read a chapter of a book. Ask for help to enable you to get this time if you need to. Other people might not think to ask you what you need. Don't be afraid to ask, most people are always happy to help!

Of course, many new mothers don't want to be away from their new baby for even a second. There is no right or wrong answer here. If you want only 5 minutes to yourself, then make sure that you get those 5 minutes. If you want a warm bubble bath for half an hour and a book, then make sure that you make that happen whenever possible. Sometimes asking for the help is hard. But you are just as important as your baby.

4

THE FIRST 40 DAYS

You might have heard of 'The First 40 Days'. You will find a few books written on this and I strongly encourage you to explore this fully and find a book that you feel fully aligned to.

Essentially, the first forty days refer literally to the 40 days after a woman has given birth. In society today, many women are expected to just 'bounce back'.... into their clothes, routines, childcare, sometimes even their jobs, while their body is still healing.

It refers to a traditional way of caring for a new mother, allowing her to rest, to remain at home and focus on her newborn child. To allow her body to start to heal, for breastfeeding to become established, for bonding to occur – without the need to rush back to her previous role.

Stay in bed, get nourishing food brought to you, watch copious amounts of Netflix documentaries, whatever makes you feel good and allows you to rest. You deserve it! And your baby deserves the best version of YOU.

(A personal note – with my 4th child, my husband went back to work after just 2 weeks. We had three other children, aged 4, 3 and 18 months. My 4-year-old needed taking to and from school, and so I would pop the baby in the sling, the middle 2 in the double pram, and the eldest would walk. It was half an hour each way to school. I was exhausted. My body didn't get the chance to heal properly, and I bled heavily in the post-partum period for six weeks.

With my 5th child I got to rest totally after her birth. The older children were cared for, school runs done, food cooked for me. Total bed rest and the chance to concentrate on the newest baby. I didn't lift a finger. My post-partum bleeding lasted only 2 weeks, and I felt so much better).

5

GETTING STARTED

Getting into the mindset for Breastfeeding

There are so many ways of breastfeeding, and every mother will develop her own style. However, the basic steps are all the same and must be in place before you start adding your own variations. And your baby is born with a natural instinct to find your breast, crawl to it, and suckle. We might just need to give them a helping hand as we go. Breastfeeding is a combination of instinct, reflex, and learning.

They might be a little clumsy at first, perhaps not opening their mouth wide enough, or they might be in the wrong position to feed effectively. By practising more, you will both become accustomed to what works for you... and what doesn't. A bit like learning how to dance – you might know the steps, but practice makes it work for you!

Quiet surroundings are incredibly helpful when breastfeeding, to give you both the chance to relax, and to pay attention to each other without distraction, especially in the first two weeks. Take your time to learn, listen to your body, relax, and let your journey unfold.

So many women almost expect themselves to fail. They hear stories from friends and family, who gave their baby a bottle of formula and they started to sleep through the night. Or who gave their baby a bottle so that family members could be involved. Of how breastfeeding your baby means you are tied to them for longer, or that they'll never be independent if they rely on your for too long.

Simply look into secure attachment theories, and you will see for yourself how responding to your baby, by developing this bond with them, how holding them, sleeping next to them, and being at one with your baby, lead to strong, independent children and adults, secure in the knowledge that they are loved.

Before You Start Any Feed

Be sure that you are comfortable, relaxed and well supported. Place cushions under your arms (a V-shaped cushion is ideal), have a drink to hand, and a snack.

If you feel that you consciously need to take steps to relax, take a deep breath, feel your lungs expand, close your eyes. Even if your baby is crying, this will help. Milk production is hormone related, and being relaxed helps with the production of the milk.

If your baby is crying, take a few seconds to calm yourself, then calm your baby before you put them to your breast. It can make all the difference.

Three Important Aspects of Breastfeeding

- The way you and your baby are positioned during feeding
- How your body works to produce and release milk
- How the composition of your milk changes during a feed

Position & Posture

A good position is one where the mother and baby are both comfortable, and the baby is in the correct position to get an effective latch. It is a bit like trying to drive in the wrong position – you will soon feel uncomfortable!

Before you start, whether you are sitting up to feed, or laying down, ask yourself if you are comfortable – can you sustain a feed in this position? You should not be in a slouched position that changes the natural shape of your breast.

Why Position Matters

Getting into the correct position to feed is important for both the mother and the baby, even for those who are bottle fed. Think of how to drive a car – you cannot reach the peddles if your seat is too far back, your ankles hurt, and your shoulders hurt if you are too close. So being in a good and comfortable position is important. Of course, as your baby grows and you're both comfortable with feeding, you'll likely change your positioning.

For some women and babies, learning to breastfeed comes easily. For others it may take a bit more practice. Please do allow yourself the time that you need and try to ensure that you are able to concentrate, and can remain relaxed while you learn.

Getting Positioning Right

Your posture - being comfortable is key – your back, head, shoulders, neck, and arms. You need to be in a position where you can hold your baby's body close to you, and up high enough so that you don't have to lean forward to get your breast in to their mouth.

Sit up with your arms supported. A v-shaped cushion is great for this, possibly with an additional cushion under the arm that will support your baby's head. This will help you to remain comfortable, and for your breast to remain in their natural position (i.e., not hanging forward, or flattened by leaning backward). Of course, you are likely to give your baby their first feed while laying back, which is fine for that first feed.

The key to remember is that you will be bringing the baby *to* your breast, and not the other way round.

Some positions that work well include:

- Sitting on your sofa, v-cushion across your tummy and under your arm. Feet flat on the floor. Try to put a cushion at the base of your back also to help you to keep your back straight and supported.
- Laying on your side – this is a great position for when your baby has just been born and you might be sore vaginally or have a c-section wound. Lay on your side, with one hand under your head, and the other hand holding your baby close to you (please see The Lullaby Trust's guidelines for safe co-sleeping –

https://www.lullabytrust.org.uk/safer-sleep-advice).
Try to avoid distorting the natural shape of your breast if possible.

Try out different ways that make you feel comfortable, and that allow for you not to lean back, or distort the natural shape of your breasts. Use cushions or pillows to support your arms and back, have water and snacks to hand.

Avoid breastfeeding in a rush, to make sure that you get your positioning right, to allow you to maintain that position in comfort for the duration of the feed.

Once you and your baby have got your breastfeeding journey off to a good start, you will be able to feed while doing other things if you want to!

How to hold your baby

Once you are comfortable, you need to hold your baby in a good position for them to be able to breastfeed. They must be comfortable, supported and close to you.

- Hold your baby with their body facing toward you, so that you don't have to turn their head. Your nipple should be in line with their nose, and not their mouth. Their entire body should be supported from head to bottom, though refrain from pulling their head to your breast. Use your arms and hands to support your baby, with pillows under your arms to keep you comfortable and prevent neck, shoulder, and back strain.

- Your baby should be nose to nipple. They will smell your milk and will open their mouth. Having their nose in line with your nipple means that they will have to open their mouth wide, enabling a deeper latch.

- Their head, neck and back should be in almost a straight line. Their head should not be tilted down, and should not be turned towards you, but rather their body facing you – a good position never requires your baby to turn their head to feed when they are so young.

You may find that your baby prefers feeding on one side rather than the other. Many women breastfeed very successfully from just one breast, so while you should always offer both breasts in the early days, please do not allow it to become a source of stress (which will in turn reduce milk production!)

In summary, make sure that:

- You are comfortable
- Your baby is well supported
- Your baby is held close to you
- Your baby is turned toward you
- Your baby is nose to nipple
- Your baby has their head, neck and back in a straight line
- Their arms and hands do not get in the way (the lower arm should be hanging beneath them – you may need to tuck it up but it should not be in the way)

Avoid:

- Allowing your baby's chin to push against your breast
- Laying your baby on their back so that they need to turn their head to feed
- Bringing your breast to your baby – bring your baby to your breast

In some women, especially those with larger breasts, it may be necessary for them to hold their breast. This is best done by holding the breast from underneath, and avoiding changing the shape of the breast. Once baby is latched comfortably, you may be able to remove the hand holding your breast. There is no harm in remaining in that position if required/preferred.

How your baby takes your breast

The principles for how your baby will take your breast are the same for all babies. It requires time, patience, and a relaxing environment. Putting pressure on yourself to feed (or pressure from others) can often be counter-productive and affect your breast-feeding journey. As previously mentioned, surround yourself with people who will support your desire for breastfeeding.

Family Support

You might be surprised by how many people are set in their own ways and have beliefs around breastfeeding, without them even knowing where these thoughts have come from. Make sure that your family know of your plan to breastfeed and make it clear that you would like their support. Ensure that they know that if you want advice that you will ask for it, and perhaps suggest that they read up on breastfeeding themselves.

What to do if breastfeeding hurts

You will hear that if breastfeeding hurts then you are doing it wrong. This isn't strictly true. Yes, pain can come from an incorrect latch. If this happens, stop the feed (you can release the suction by slipping a clean finger into the corner of their mouth, and remove your nipple from their mouth), and then try again.

But the early days may feel uncomfortable, especially as breastfeeding can help the womb to shrink back to pre-baby size, often known as after-pains. If pain only lasts for a few seconds, then it is like going as it should. But pain for longer than that indicates an issue.

If you are certain that positioning is correct, and that the latch is fine, it would be worth getting your baby checked for tongue tie. If severe, it may need cutting.

Signs that your baby is feeding well

- Your baby should have opened their mouth wide, and taken a large mouthful of breast (not just nipple)

- Their lower lip should be in contact with the areola, surrounding the nipple and not just pinching

- The tip of their nose can be touching your breast, but not squashed. Baby's noses are biologically designed to allow them to breathe while feeding, so do not feel that you need to pull them away from your breast

- Their bottom lip should be turned back against your breast. You will feel the sensation of their tongue and jaw almost drawing the milk from your mouth

- At the beginning of a feed, your baby will take some quick sucks. This will soon progress to stronger, deep, rhythmic sucks. You might feel the 'let down' which can feel like a tingling feeling in _both_ breasts. The opposite breast may leak! Do not be surprised by this as it is totally normal. Your baby will likely suck a few times, pause, then suck again.

- Your baby will continue to feed quite happily until they decide that they have finished.

- Feeding should not be painful for you. If it is on occasion, release your baby's latch and try again

When your baby has finished with one breast, offer them the other if you feel that you need to/they are still hungry. Do not worry if they are too tired or full to try. Some babies only ever feed off one breast per feed!

Milk Supply and How It Is Released

This is a two-part relationship, where your body is working to get your milk and its composition right.

During pregnancy, pregnancy hormones prepared your body for making milk, especially the colostrum required in the early days.

These hormones also limit the amount of milk made when your baby is first born, as their tummies are very small. As soon as your baby is born, the hormone *prolactin* is release, to start your breasts on producing a generous milk supply.

When you put your baby to your breast, and they start to suckle, your brain reads the message that your breasts need to make milk to replace what the baby is taking. It is a constant cycle of

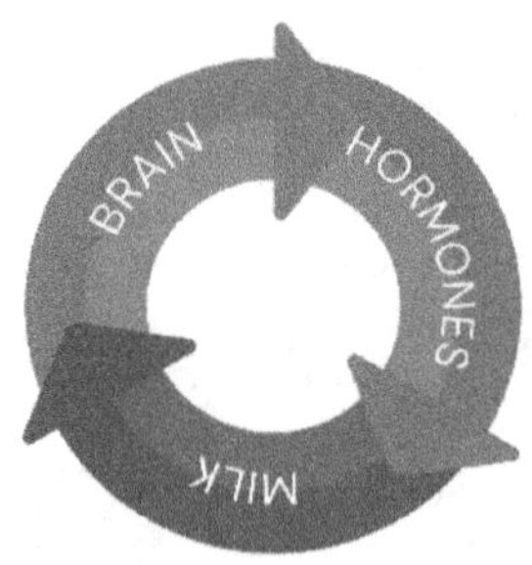

It truly is supply and demand, although it feels more fitting to say demand and supply!

Make sure that you offer your breasts regularly and your baby feeds well, especially in those early days and weeks while your supply is becoming established. Bad positioning, or not allowing your baby to feed enough will ultimately result in your breasts not making enough milk – they simply won't receive the brain signals adequately.

After producing the milk in your breasts, your breasts need to release it. Milk is released due to the let-down reflex, and your baby feeding well.

You might even find that simply hearing your baby causes your let-down reflex. You might feel it as a tingle in your breasts, sometimes bordering on a light stinging type of sensation. You might also find that it happens if your baby is *due* a feed. You may even experience let-down when you hear another baby cry!

You may find that in the first few days after giving birth that your womb contracts and is painful when you feed. This is perfectly normal and is due to the oxytocin being released.

Oxytocin is the hormone responsible for the let-down, for the contractions in labour, and is also released during lovemaking. The function of the womb contractions following birth is to help clear your womb of blood. It is a healthy process that your body goes through.

These contractions also help your womb to go back to its pre-baby size more quickly, which can be what causes the afterpains. You may find that the afterpains are more painful the more children you have, as your womb contractions need to work harder to reduce its size. These feelings should only last for a couple of days.

Oxytocin tends not to be released in stressful situations, which can impact milk production. Trying to stay relaxed during feeds, and not stress about the feeding itself, should help to prevent this from happening. Some women do find themselves in a circle of stress where the baby is struggling to latch, Mum stresses, Mum is uncomfortable, baby continues to cry, cause more stress, resulting in slower milk production due to the inhibition of oxytocin.

Breaking the cycle is key. Relax as much as you can before and during the feed. Don't be tempted to rush, or you will end up feeling you haven't done well or satisfied your baby. This feeling, if felt too often, can lead to the end of your journey.

Getting yourself comfortable, and your baby latched well, should hopefully lead to a relaxed and comforting feed for you both.

If you do find that you are struggling to relax, a warm flannel placed on your breast, or nipple stimulation may be enough to stimulate a let-down.

The composition of your breast milk is never the same. The milk (colostrum) in the first few days is different from milk at 2 weeks old. At 2 weeks it is different from at 3 months, which is again different at 1 year.

Every mother produces milk that is suited to their own baby. If your baby were to develop a cold for example, your milk would change to give them the antibodies that they need to fight it. **Isn't that wonderful?!** By them suckling, or by you kissing their head, your body works to make them better.

Milk composition also changes *during* a feed. At the beginning of the feed, you may find that you get a lot of milk flowing quickly. This used to be referred to as foremilk, lower in fat and higher in quantity, with hindmilk (milk at the later part of the feed) being the opposite. This is outdated information now, but something that is still referred to, and you may hear it mentioned during your breastfeeding journey.

The La Leche League states:

" as milk is made, fat sticks to the sides of the milk-making cells and the watery part of the milk moves down the ducts towards your nipple, where it mixes with any milk left there from the last feed. The longer the time between feeds, the more diluted the leftover milk becomes. This 'watery' milk has a higher lactose content and less fat than the milk stored in the milk-making cell further into your breast.

You can't tell how much fat your baby has received from the length of a feed. Some babies take a full feed in five minutes, while others take 40 minutes to get the same amount. As long as your baby is breastfeeding effectively, you can let them decide how long to feed for, and they will get all the fat that they need "

The change in milk composition happens naturally during the feed, and it is essential that your baby feeds for long enough to get both types of milk. Do not remove your baby from your breast mid-feed. Your baby will know when they are full, as their baby sense the relevant signals. So you just need to let your baby feed when they are hungry, and let the stay nursing until they come off themselves. You can then offer the second breast, but they might not want it. You could burp your baby in between switching if you would like to. Some babies will always accept the second breast while others might never need it. At the next feed, offer the second breast (from the current feed) first.

Some women wear a special bracelet to remind them which breast to feed from next time, or a hairband on your wrist, or even twist the clasp of your breastfeeding bra to know which breast is next. You might even be able to tell from the size and feel of your breast.

By not limiting the amount of time that your baby has at the breast, you can feel confident that they are getting what they need.

Having set times between feeds and believing that a baby is manipulating you by crying and that you shouldn't give in, are all very outdated thoughts. Research has progressed but society has not. Feed your baby on demand – you *cannot* feed a breastfed baby too much.

Over time, the length of each feed will change as they get older, and the composition will too. If you find your baby seems to need feeding more often, it might simply be a growth spurt. Don't get into the way of thinking that you aren't producing enough milk – **you are**! Your baby just knows how to stimulate your breasts to make more milk.

Having said this, breaking off a baby's feed occasionally won't affect your journey. Sometimes all they need is a quick top up before getting in the car. You don't need to be sat around for hours at a time. Though in the early days, this **is** essential so that you get feeding established and you get to rest.

6

BREASTFEEDING ISSUES

Inverted, and flat nipples

Inverted nipples are those that dip inward, rather than straight out. Flat nipples are those that do not stand out when a woman is cold, aroused, or starting to breastfeed.

It *is* possible to breastfeed, it just might take a little longer or be a little more difficult to start.

But **please** remember - babies **breast** feed, not nipple feed! They need to take in a large mouthful of breast. Doing so should draw the nipple out when they suckle.

It can sometimes be useful for a woman to stimulate their nipples, and to gently express a small amount of milk to the end of their nipple, to encourage their baby to suckle.

Relactating

For some women, their breastfeeding journey might end, even when they didn't want it to. They might then decide to try breastfeeding again.

Or perhaps your baby is unwell and you'd like to give them the best nourishment again?

Or have tried formula and is hasn't agreed with your baby.

Whatever the reasons to try, many women are able to re-start their milk supply. To start breastfeeding again, spend time having skin to skin with your baby, and regularly offer them your breast, as often as you can, and for as long as you can. Ensure a good position for you both and have patience.

It is a good idea to replace just one bottle feed to start with, at the same kind of time each day. Your body will soon start to recognise these regular cues, and you can build up from there.

Problems with breastfeeding and feelings around it

When women experience problems with breastfeeding, it is a deep rooted, emotional feeling. It can cause a woman upset that she didn't expect to experience.

This can often be made worse by partners, family, or friends who don't support your desire to breastfeed. Who may suggest that <u>you</u> are the problem, or the baby is. They might try to push the idea of formula and bottles, which you simply might not want to do.

These feelings can put stress on your relationship with your partner, and even with the bond with your baby.

The easiest thing in this situation is to place blame. It might not be a conscious thought. It could be you being blamed; you could blame baby!

But remember!!

** Problems can almost always be solved. And will always have a cause **

Do not blame yourself..... you haven't done anything wrong.

Do not blame your baby. They are not being demanding, doing this on purpose, being aggressive, or manipulating you. They are, quite simply, **being a baby**.

Do not blame your body. Women's bodies are designed to breastfeed!

Chances are that the problem that you are experiencing are down to:

- Positioning
- Latch

Try to relax, breathe deeply.... you've GOT THIS!! Go back through the basics. Relax. Sit comfortably. Support yourself and your baby. Make sure your baby is positioned so that they have to open their mouth wide to take in more of your breast in to their mouth. Work on getting the latch right.

YOU ARE AMAZING! PLEASE REMEMBER THAT!

Breast Issues

Some women find that they experience pain or inflammation in their breasts.

Engorgement – this often happens when milk 'comes in', during the 2nd to 4th days following birth (typically, though it may be longer following a caesarean section). It can happen at other times too, before milk supply settles down, or if your baby goes for longer between feeds. Breasts can become swollen and painful, often hard to the touch. It is usually a sign that milk is not flowing effectively from the breast.

This might be due to:

- Baby's positioning
- Not feeding frequently enough
- Not feeding for long enough

Feeding frequently and for as long as your baby wants to can fix engorgement. You may need to gently hand express before a feed, if you feel that your breasts are too full to allow your baby to latch well.

If you have relief from the pressure between feeds, gentle hand expression can help, as can using a warm flannel, or having a warm shower. This hand expression is not the same as using a pump to express (which would encourage further supply). But a gentle pressure and stroking of the breasts to encourage milk to flow. It can offer instant relief. You should find that you are then able to feed your baby.

Mastitis

Mastitis is indicated by red, inflamed breasts, that are sometimes hot to the touch if infected and the normal flow of milk is restricted.

It is more likely to occur when the normal flow of feeding is disturbed (by returning to work for example).

Common signs of mastitis are:

- A painful area within the breast
- A red area that is hot to touch
- You may have chills and shivers
- You may have flu-like symptoms

If you start to have these feelings, it is important to start treatment immediately by:

- Feeding your baby often, and for as long as they want
- Gently massage any lumpy of blocked areas that you can feel or see (using an electric toothbrush can be effective)
- Be careful with the positioning of your baby
- Try to hand express some milk to relieve pressure along with breastfeeding
- Drink plenty of water and REST!
- You may need to contact your doctor to be treated with antibiotics.

Avoiding feeding your baby will simply make matters worse.

Continue to feed, making sure that position and latch are correct. Trying different positions to allow the breast to be drained away from the infected area. For example, holding the baby tucked under your arm.

If these steps do not start to relieve your symptoms, please contact your doctor as it may be infected.

Blocked Ducts

Blocked ducts occur when the breast milk is not flowing well. It shouldn't be painful. You may feel lumps in your breast.

Blocked ducts usually indicate that positioning of the baby needs to be improved, and trying out different positions can be useful. For example, laying down to feed, feeding with baby tucked under your armpit, feeding with baby across your front. Feed from the lumpy side first as the initial stronger suction at the start of the feed will likely be much more efficient at unblocking the duct.

Sore Nipples

A large number of women find that at the start of breastfeeding, their nipples become sore. However, this is not something that should be accepted as the norm. It is almost always a sign that your baby isn't latched or positioned correctly, causing nipple damage.

The main cure for sore nipples is to get the positioning of the baby right. That strong suction at the beginning of a feed will cause pain if incorrectly latched. It is fine to remove your baby from your breast as many times as needed to get the latch correct and pain free.

Please do not be tempted to stop feeding without solving the positioning problem as the pain will come back again.

Some women resort to nipple shields or creams, but these *do not* solve the actual problem, though you may some short term relief while using them. If you do want to put something on your nipples, then breastmilk and air work best. Sore nipples heal fast once positioning is right. Do not avoid feeding your baby during this time, or you risk engorgement, and even possible mastitis.

Tongue Tie and Lip Tie

Some babies are born with a tongue tie, and others with a lip tie, which should be diagnosed at post-birth checks. In some cases, if severe, the tie can impact breastfeeding and may need cutting. Contacting your midwife, health visitor or doctor should get you a referral, or some practitioners offer private services. It is a simple and quick procedure, and your baby will be able to feed immediately after.

Not Having Enough Milk

Only 1% of women (a bit less actually) are actually unable to produce enough milk to feed their babies.

If women were unable to produce enough milk, if it wasn't enough for their babies, if it caused tooth decay and any number of other suggested 'issues' with breastmilk, then the human race would have died out years before artificial milk was invented!

Unfortunately, society today has promoted artificial milk, and sexualised breasts so much, to the point that women feel like they're failing. The second that they mention that their baby feeds often, or isn't sleeping through the night (most adults don't sleep through the night!), they often have formula and bottles suggested to them as a solution. Not to mention that women are told that breastfeeding their baby after a certain age is 'wrong' due to the sexualisation of breasts.

If a woman is found to be having issues with breastfeeding, it is most likely that it is a positioning and latch issue, rather than a supply issue.

If you don't feel supported in your breastfeeding journey, please do contact a lactation specialist for support.

Remember: your body makes as much milk as is needed, and it is made on demand. The milk composition is designed perfectly for your baby. Supplementing with formula can be extremely damaging to your breastfeeding journey, as you will produce less milk. Plus, you risk initial engorgement.

This is also why feeds should not be timed. Be led by your baby. Timing feeds can mean that your breast is not fully empty, and therefore less will be produced to 'fill' it again.

Oversupply

Some women find that they have an oversupply of milk, especially in the early days once milk has 'come in'. This is normal in the first week, as the milk is produced and isn't only producing the amount needed. After the first week or two it should calm down.

If the oversupply continues beyond the first week, it may be due to your baby being taken off the breast too soon at a feed, in order to offer them the other breast. So they haven't fully emptied the breast effectively.

Symptoms of oversupply are:

- Breasts that are full and tender between feeds (even after feeding is established)
- You leak milk, causing your clothing to be regularly wet (you may find that you leak from the opposite breast during a feed which is normal).
- Your baby pulls away during a feed, spluttering and choking
- Your baby gains weight very fast
- Your baby brings up more than a couple of mouthfuls after most feeds

Before taking any potential action, it is worth giving it a couple of weeks to see if your supply settles on its own. You can gently hand express to relieve uncomfortable 'fullness'.

If you know that your baby is well latched, you might consider feeding from one breast completely per feed, rather than offering the second breast.

Please know that your baby knows instinctively what they are doing:

How to feed

How long to feed for

When to stop feeding

You simply need to ensure that for your breastfeeding journey to get off to a good start, and to continue positively, that ensuring an effective latch, and being comfortable and rested yourself, are key elements.

Women are designed to breastfeed. Our breasts, our hormones, all lead to us being able to do this magical thing for our children. Each mother is unique, her breastmilk is unique and made exclusively for her baby.

When her baby is unwell, her breastmilk creates antibodies delivered via the milk to make her baby well. It changes as the baby goes through the day, as her baby gets older, and is the perfect nourishment for her baby.

7

LACTOSE OVERLOAD AND CMPI

Lactose Overload

(Previously referred to as hindmilk/foremilk imbalance)

Some women, especially those with an oversupply, may find that their baby suffers additional symptoms to suggest a lactose overload.

Symptoms may include:

- Growing well but not content
- Pulling away from the breast
- Crying inconsolably just after or between feeds
- Having wet, frothy, yellow or green explosive stools

You can help your baby by:

- Establishing a deeper latch
- Trying different feeding positions, especially one laying down
- Try offering feeds more frequently, to allow your baby to have more manageable feeds, rather than larger feeds spaced out

The amount of lactose in your milk is not a result of your diet. Lactose is a carbohydrate that needs to be broken down for it to be absorbed. When your baby is drinking large amounts of breastmilk, it is easy to see why their body might struggle to break it down. This is not an allergy to cow's milk in your diet, but rather a digestion issue. It is not necessary to reduce the amount of cow's milk in your diet.

Cow's Milk Protein Intolerance (CMPI)

This is a sensitivity to protein in cow's milk that a mother may be consuming, but it is not a lactose intolerance. These particular proteins are molecules passed from mother to baby through her milk, which may not be broken down effectively due to their size. Your baby may be more sensitive to these proteins, and if so may display the following symptoms:

- Wheezing
- Vomiting
- Diarrhoea
- Blood in stools
- Constipation
- Eczema
- A rash
- Blocked nose

If CMPI is suspected due to these symptoms, then cutting out dairy products from your own diet for a number of weeks might help you to see a change in your baby. Many babies do grow out of this sensitivity to the cow's milk protein.

8

THE ACCEPTANCE OF BOTTLES

The Acceptance of Bottles

Unfortunately, due to breasts being overtly sexualised by the media, a huge number of people are uncomfortable with seeing breasts in public. Many women are asked to cover their breasts when feeding in public or told that they can feed in a toilet cubicle, not at the table.

There are many subconscious symbols around us that promotes bottle feeding, even from a young age.

Think of all those toy babies that come with a bottle?

How feeding rooms in airports and shopping centres often use a bottle image as an indication of the use of the room?

We have been made to believe that we must know the exact amounts of milk that our baby should be getting, only possible by using bottles. Yet if we feed on demand, our baby will get the right amount. We just need to make sure that positioning, latch and comfort are at the forefront of our minds.

It isn't really any wonder that rates of breastfeeding are so low, when bottle feeding is considered the norm from when we are children. Especially if we haven't grown up seeing any/many women breastfeed. And this includes me too. A man who is understanding of breastfeeding and is able to fully support the mother of his child, can be a key element in a successful breastfeeding journey. Men can bond with their baby in so many ways that do not involve breastfeeding.

9

MODERN MYTHS

" You must prepare your nipples in pregnancy ready for breastfeeding "

- When a latch is correct, and deep, nipples should not become damaged as there won't be any friction caused inside the baby's mouth

" You must breastfeed your baby immediately after birth or you won't be able to breastfeed successfully "

- While the ideal time to breastfeed is within the first couple of hours after birth, not doing so will not affect your breastfeeding journey. Baby might simply be too tired. Plenty of skin to skin IS important however, if possible. If you are separated from your baby, you may be providing with a breastpump to get milk production started until you can feed your baby yourself

" You must time your baby's feeds "

- No. Babies are designed to feed on demand. Offer them your breast regularly

" *Babies must feed from both breasts at each feed* "

- Babies should be allowed to decide. If they refuse your offer of feeding at the second breast, then please do not force the issue.

" *Breastfed babies need water* "

- Your baby gets everything that they need from you, so water is not necessary.

" *Feeding a baby for longer means they get more milk* "

- Each baby has their own rate of feeding, and each woman releases milk at her own rate. So timing is not an indication of the amount of milk taken

" *Nipples should be healed by the use of nipple shields, creams, resting her nipples, stopping breastfeeding* "

- The _cause_ of the problem needs addressing, usually the latch. Not feeding, or resting your nipples may affect the supply (as baby won't be encouraging the supply by feeding) and the use of shields and creams simply mask the issue, which will still be there when you stop using them

" *You've fed before! You must know what you're doing?* "

- Every baby is different, every journey is different. These kind of comments can be extremely detrimental to a woman's mental health surrounding breastfeeding.

" *Women with engorged breasts should not express milk to relieve them* "

- Gentle hand expression to provide relief is fine. But do not use a pump as this will encourage engorgement

" *Young babies cry a lot and should be left to cry* "

- Developing a secure attachment with your baby is the best thing to do. They need to know you are there, in the same way that adults need love and affection! Babies simply don't know how to express themselves in any other way. A sling is a great way to encourage this bonding process. By creating this early bond, you are paving the way to a wonderful relationship in the future

" You will spoil your baby if you are always giving her what she wants "

- You cannot spoil a baby. You are simply responding to their needs. They need cuddles, rocking and feeding to sleep. To feel comforted and close to you. After all, you are their world

"Breastfeeding hurts. It is just something that everyone has to put up with "

- If breastfeeding is going well, and the latch is good, then it shouldn't hurt. Ongoing pain is a sign that something is wrong. It should not be expected, or something to be ignored, or excused. In the first few days, there may be a short, sharp pain during the first few seconds of the latch, but it should not last long, and certainly not throughout the feed

" Your milk is too thick/too thin "

- Your milk is exactly what your baby needs. There is no such thing as too thin or too thick. Just let your baby feed for as long as they need, and as often as they need

Further resources:

Free eBook guide to baby growth spurts

https://bit.ly/freegrowthspurtebook

Join our Facebook group here:

www.facebook.com/groups/thebreastfeedingacademy

La Leche League GB

https://www.laleche.org.uk/

La Leche League International

https://llli.org/

The Breastfeeding Network

https://www.breastfeedingnetwork.org.uk/

The Association of Breastfeeding Mothers

https://abm.me.uk/

ABOUT THE AUTHOR

Thank you so much for purchasing this book. It has been a real labour of love as a Mum working around a toddler every day, and worth every minute.

I am hugely passionate about helping women to have the breastfeeding journey that they want, on their terms. But with breastfeeding support, education and knowledge so low, it isn't really any wonder that breastfeeding rates are so low.

I have breastfed 7 children myself, and know the struggles when you are not feeling supported or educated.

I truly hope that this book makes a difference in your journey
~ Deborah ~